Anti Aging

Anti Dis-ease

Booklet

ANTI-AGING

ANTI-DIS-EASE

BY: Freddie Martin Arbuthnot

Contents (just guidelines, Not organized well enough for real contents)

Introduction

Treating Chronic Disease

Learning and Giving

Some things to Avoid

Supplements

New Chapter

Some Favorite Things

Life Happenings

More Learning

Experts

Questions??

More Life Coaching

Anti-Aging/Anti-dis-ease

By Freddie Martin Arbuthnot

These little booklets that I write are written to dispense the information that I am learning. I was born in 1934 and have been learning new stuff from the day I was born and for the past 15 years I have had a passion for telling others what I am learning. I grew up in the country with a great family and many of the things that I learned on the farm continues to be a large part of my wellness program.

When I went into Nursing school and became a registered nurse 1955, many of the things that I learned were not different from the things that I grew up knowing, that soon changed as the drug companies took charge of our health care and greed took over. As I worked as a nurse, I became so agitated with the drugs, the physicians and insurance companies my job as a nurse became very tiring. I worked in hospital, administration of nursing facilities, industry. and almost every position in healthcare. Over the years everything has become even worse, so I retired early and became as educated as possible in holistic/alternative healing. I continue to learn every day.

My husband died in 1980 from brain cancer with all the "medical" modalities, he was blind for a year before his death, and I had 4 children to get through high school and college. I worked 3 jobs at a time to make enough money and feel that every job, had some good things to teach me. Here is a partial list: Mary Kay Beauty Consultant, Real Estate sales, Personnel director and nurse for a factory, Breakfast manager for hotel, Photo lab tech for 1 hour photo, Bear builder, retail sales, Pampered Chef consultant, desk clerk for hotel, Administrator of medical care facility, Director of nursing for nursing home, Nursing manager Rehab facility, Employment counsellor, private nursing, investigating claims in Insurance office of large corp. real estate sales. Special Events planer, caterer, and pet sitter. I may have left out a few jobs, but I learned a lot in all these jobs and when I made a change, written on my exit interview was always "good for rehire". I never burn a bridge, I may have to walk that bridge again.

When I retired, I kept working because my social security check has stayed between $800 and $900, I now work, doing wellness life planning and teaching classes on wellness. I do not charge for my services but take donations. I live with a dozen rescued dogs, a couple of cats, a couple of really, elderly pigmy goats and a senior horse, 36 years old. We laugh and play and live healthy lives, I have used my medicare card for an eye injury but have never taken a prescribed medication or an "over the counter' drug. My animals never need a vet either, listening to my body *and treating with holistic modalities has been very successful for me and my animals.*

I consider myself a connector, I love to connect people to people who can assist them in their wellness journey I never forget my father walking on the farm and pulling up a beet as he says, "sister eat plenty of these, they keep your blood healthy", he was also reminding me often that we must care for others and help someone else, every day.

It is my hope that the information in this little book will be helpful in the life of everyone who reads it.

I self-publish these little booklets, therefore it is written in my language and there will be some mistakes. Take in the information and forget the mistakes. I learn new tidbits and immediately want to share the information so humor me and READ IT!

Treating Chronic Disease

Some suggestions for treatment of chronic disease (cancer)

- ✓ *Be certain that your water is pure and never become thirsty*
- ✓ *Breathe pure air*

- ✓ *Bathe or do foot bath of hot water with Epson salt added or Dead Sea Salt, do this at least 3 times a week*
- ✓ *Think positive thoughts and laugh and play many times a day*
- ✓ *Take a good multi vitamin like Moringa every day, I believe in real food, moringa is a plant, I seldom take a supplement that is composed of a few chemicals put together.*
- ✓ *Drink a glass of water with 1 teaspoon of diatomaceous earth every morning on an empty stomach*
- ✓ *Black seed oil 1 teaspoonful morning and evening or 2 capsules. When you study black seed oil, you will read that there are at least 101 reasons to use black cumin seed oil*
- ✓ *Put your feet and hands on the earth, walk barefoot or work in the dirt with your hands, earth's energy is so very healing and it is given to us, FREE. We can all benefit from using this energy to heal all parts of our body, mind and soul.*
- ✓ *Get lots of sunshine, if you are not getting enough sunshine, you cannot heal, most healers believe that almost everyone is deficient in vitamin D and that many health problems can be traced directly to this problem. If you are not getting sunshine, as an alternative, you can take it in supplement form.*
- ✓ *Swish and swallow Noni juice every day, about an ounce. This fruit is a must have for everyone, in my opinion. What noni does for our wellness is amazing.*

- ✓ *Rub frankincense oil on area of tumors, etc. 3 times a day, other oils can be used but I think this one is the best. It would be great if we all studied our essential oils and made use of them.*
- ✓ *Alpha lipoic acid at least twice a day, I must also add information on,*
- ✓ *Cordyceps: cell healer, if you state a body part, cordyceps increases it's wellness; blood sugar normalized, heart health, lungs/respiratory wellness, immune system, if you want to build your immune system, this is the supplement/food, kidney support/healing,, I have heard testimonials that this with some dietary changes can keep people off dialysis. In my opinion we should all add this supplement to our healing protocol. When I was teaching from a health food store, the testimonials kept coming about this mushroom*
- ✓ *Pectasol or citrus pectin daily, if you are not having at least 2 bms a day. If we ate an organic apple every day, we would never need this product.*
- ✓ *Fermented foods and drinks*
- ✓ *Sprouted foods*
- ✓ *B17 and Paw Paw as directed on the bottle, if your diagnosis is cancer.*
- ✓ *Rub on Magnesium 3 times a day*
- ✓ *If available, drink goat milk kefir before each meal, 2 ounces*

- ✓ *Put on your food lots of ginger, garlic, turmeric, black pepper*
- ✓ *Use lots of good bone broth in your meals and eat lots of fresh vegetables*
- ✓ *Rhodiola, Ashwanganda and Ginseng, one capsule morning and evening. These herbs are wonderful adaptogens and can really be beneficial with your mood.*
- ✓ *Weekly massage, if possible*
- ✓ *If available go to a colonic therapist and get enemas several times*
- ✓ *I know that I have missed a few things but this is a start, I would say that the most important thing is: Laugh, sing, hum, whistle, play and have fun every day.*

Dementia/ Alzheimer's

- ✓ *Read books on curing Alzheimer disease: I think Peggy Sarlin has the best one and I can give you others*
- ✓ *Coconut oil every 4-6 hours, I like Brain Octain by Bulletproof.com*
- ✓ *Ashwanganda, Rhodiola. Ginseng, or other mood builders because most dementia sufferers are depressed*
- ✓ *Ketogenic nutrition program because brain does better burning ketones instead of carbs.*
- ✓ *Lots of sunshine and earthing*
- ✓ *Great nutrition and supplements*
- ✓ *Filtered structured water and clean air*
- ✓ *Black seed oil*

- ✓ *Be active*
- ✓ *Keep blood sugar under control with supplements and nutrition*
- ✓ *Chemical free personal care products, no fluoride.*
- ✓ *Kefir, I prefer Goat milk kefir.*
- ✓ *I would never, never, never take the prescription drug that are on the market at this time.*
- ✓ *New natural healing modalities become available every day, so seek out an alternative medicine person for information and read about the natural treatments.*

If you have a problem with metabolic syndrome (type two diabetes) most experts will say that it can be easily cured if you water and broth fast for several days and go on the ketogenic program, you will reset your metabolism.

Some aches and pains will go away if you go on a completely grain free nutrition program and do a three day bone broth fast.

Learning and Giving

I am confident that there is nothing in life that replaces the effort to learn new things all the time. I have now past my 83rd birthday and I am even more determined to learn new things every day and also to spend my life helping others, I want to make someone's life better every day that I live. If I had a motto it would be this old hymn:

Have I done any good in the world today

Have I helped anyone in need

Have I cheered up the sad

And made someone feel glad?

If not I have failed indeed

Has anyone's burden been lighter today

Because I was willing to share?

Have the sick and the weary

Been helped on their way?

When they needed my help, was I there?

There are other verses and I would encourage you to look it up on www.youtube.com *and make it your motto.*

Some suggestions of good deeds, some cost and some don't: help at the animal shelter, make a stew or chili for a homeless shelter, offer rides to homeless to a shelter, pay lunch fees for school children, give college student a gift card to the book store, pay for someone's fill up at the service station, pay toll fee for people behind you, give transportation tokens to people without automobile, find people in a nursing home who have no relatives and become a friend, take week of groceries to poor family, collect things and money for Salvation Army, help jobless get a job, assist with community garden, help immigrants learn English, provide transportation for people to get to their job, assist with meals on wheels program, assist with groups who provide food for the unemployed and poor, connect people who can help each other, visit the homebound people and do little things to make them happy, provide a massage for a homebound person or a wheelchair bound nursing home resident, connect poor and homeless with haircuts, I could list a million things but would run out of space. Use y our imagination and think about what the needs are, Just do it!

This week another live streaming conference on curing cancer, new information on humming as a healing modality, more information on the effect of forgiveness on our wellness, new cures with goat milk kefir, new ways to unclutter my life, new information on helping people who have trouble sleeping, etc., etc.

Today I decided that I must write on the blog more often and will stop looking at facebook, as it has become toxic for me. The store I have been working from is closing so I am also looking for new venues in which to teach a class and will start in a classroom in First Christian Church in Rogers and also look for opportunities, anytime, anywhere.

I have become really fond of Audible and it has made learning much easier as I can listen to many of the books that I am trying to read. You 2.0, Hear your body whisper, Unclutter your mind, Unlimited Memory, Headstrong, Mind over Medicine, Human Heart Cosmic Heart, and many, many more.

I have many new books on Kindle but these Audibles are so much easier to just listen and learn. Some books I have to purchase in paperback because I must share them with others. The book: Drug grabbers had to be purchase so I could have it handy for others to use. When people keep taking prescriptions, I have to make them aware of the things that are being deleted from their bodies, so they can replace them.

I use a modified Ketogenic nutrition program and because I live alone I depend on Dr. Cowan's vegetable powder to provide a lot of my nutrition. I can eat an egg, add vegetable powder and have 8 vegetables in my meal without purchasing all those vegetables that will waste away in my refrigerator. I do depend upon my goat milk and goat milk kefir daily, my fruits are some powdered noni, mangosteen, gogi berry added to some goat milk, bone broth powder a little honey, black seed oil and coconut oil. I never get through the day without moringa as my multivitamin, mineral supplement. Diatomaceous earth is another supplement that I think is necessary for most people. If you are taking prescription drugs or over the counter drugs, you must take many more supplements. Stretching and rebounding and other exercise is an important part of the wellness program, especially rebounding and stretching. I consume: raw milk, moderate amounts of grass fed meats, at least 3 cups or coffee every day, and on accession, I have my onion rings and cake and ice cream. You may not be able to do this but, my body tolerates these things well, in moderation.

The number one thing you can do for your wellness; laugh, sing/hum and have fun every day. If you learn to listen to your body, you can be much better equipped to handle all your problems.

Sometimes your chronic illness can be "cured" with becoming hydrated, drink water and add to the water 1/8 teaspoon of sea salt or Himalayan salt. You must be certain that your water is free of chloride and fluoride; they are brain killers.

If you want to learn more about heart disease or just how to live a healthy life; read the book, Human Heart, Cosmic Heart by Dr. Tom Cowan. This is a great book with really great information, I order my vegetable powders from Dr Cowan's Garden and even though they are a bit expensive, I think they are necessary for me to have a great healthy life.

I am always learning about great modalities for healing and I do my research. I have been really impressed by the possibilities for this modality for healing and want to learn more; Psych K energy healing. I, of course, spend hours learning about this modality and now have videos, audios and books to learn from. I can't find a way to learn it online and can't afford to go to the workshops so must just trust others in my circle that have learned the information. I have recently become acquainted with a company called, "Vibesup", concerning vibrational healing and I am learning more about their products.

Today I also watched a documentary: Prosperity, and really enjoyed it, I also will follow through and find things I can do to help the world become a better place and that does not mean the usa become better, it means the whole world, everything is global.

I am always amazed that even though the information on how to be well is available, most people do not read, listen and absorb the information. I repeat things over and over and over and yet it is not learned. I repeat every day about our need for lots of magnesium and that every part of our body uses it and our soil is depleted so our food does not contain it or most of our lifesaving minerals and vitamins, the information just is not absorbed. This is not dumb people it is even the most intelligent people

Because quiet often poor memory is associated with age, I have been working very hard to keep my memory and have been making use of Audio books, kindle, etc., to improve my memory. One book that I have on my kindle and in my audible books library: How to improve your memory in 30 days, De clutter your mind, Unlimited mind, Boost your brain Power, Learn like Einstein, etc. I also take several supplements that help my focus, energy, etc. Probably the number 1 thing to do is, put as little as possible refined sugars and artificial stuff in my body.

Not only my brain but as we age we must keep our muscles and joints very healthy and active, that is done by movement, any movement. If you can blend the movement and socialization, that is great. I stretch, rebound, lift, etc. every day and am usually barefoot a lot of the time. I read, hum, move, spend time in the sunshine, do something that helps someone else, touch my animals, take the supplements that my body needs, drink live filtered water, enjoy my cups of coffee and try to be certain that I get quality sleep. Dr. Norm Shealy states that, dog saliva is the best anti depression drug and has no negative side effects, and is free.

Things that I try to avoid:

- *Genetically modified food*
- *Eating from cans and boxes*
- *Microwave oven*
- *Vegetable oils*
- *Processed sugars*
- *Artificial sweeteners*
- *Self centeredness*
- *Drinking water from faucet: no fluoride water*
- *Sitting more than 30 minutes without movement or stretching*
- *Chemically laden cosmetics and personal products*
- *Highly processed food, I try not to eat from a box or a can*

16

- *Unnecessary prescription drugs or over the counter drugs*
- *Plastic containers*
- *Aluminum foil if it touches my food*
- *Vaccines, root canals, mercury tooth fillings*
- *Mammograms and x-rays (use digital only)*
- *Negative people*

It is not in my belief system to think of negatives but sometimes I do have to deal with negative things. Someone was recently reviewing a book and mentioned that he had been raised with the word "when" not, "if". So you would say, "when I get that perfect job," not if I get it.. I have been thinking about that but . I usually tell my life planning clients that I do not want to hear statements like; if only they would, he would or she would. Trying to get their mindset that everything in their life is in their hands. Do not give someone else power over your life.

While I am talking about life planning; answer some questions: are you happy with your job, are you happy with who you live with, are you happy with, where you live?. If you cannot say yes to all these questions, make some positive changes in your life or you will never be completely well. And if you have a lack of forgiveness in your life and do not live a life of gratitude, you will not ever be well. If you need help planning your life or changing direction employ a life planner.

My computer quit working for a few days and I have gotten delayed with my writing. I have been really working on my memory using a book that tells me that I can be really good in 31 days, I couldn't wait so am not dong just one lesson a day, I am doing 3 or 4. I am also really doing a lot of research in Dr. Andrew Saul's books; lots of good information in "Doctor Yourself" and Fire your doctor. He uses a great deal of mega doses of vitamins.

My love for C-Span book TV, feeds my desire to learn and on Christmas Eve, I listened to 3 books that I had to memo on my phone so I could explore getting them on Audible so I could learn. The first was the interview of Michael Lewis, what a life of inquiry and learning about s many things that are happening in the world, I listened to all 3 hours, next was the book: The last Fighter Pilot, I must get this book on kindle because the writer, in his 90's talked about "Magnificent Obession" another old favorite of mine and the promise of doing something nice for someone every day. Number 3 was the book: "Surviving America in the 21st Century" by Bruder, I immediately downloaded it on Audible.

As I read, listen and analyze these books, I think of the many things that are still in my dreams: Building organic gardens in poor neighborhoods, having a mobile grooming truck with a groomer, making the stray animals look great, feel great and have adoption shows, building resumes and life coaching sessions for the homeless and people who are rebuilding their lives, providing supplements for the poor, assisting the elderly, poor to pay bills and have some luxury in their lives, giving animals to the elderly and poor, paying for their food and care so they can benefit from that pet saliva, connecting the needy with people who can provide the needs that they have in life, provide life planning for each person who had been in jail/prison, choose a few C students and provide a college or tech school education: goodness, gracious there are so many things I would like to do and to think that there are rich people who could do it all with one day of earnings. I am a socialist, I think.

The store that I am using to see clients and teach classes has gone out of business so I am going to start a new chapter in my life, finding another place to use for my classes. The store employees are also starting new chapters in their lives and I am trying to help as much as I can. Because the store is now selling all the supplements for 50% off, I have purchased many, many bottles of supplements for friends and family and many for future use.

Supplements

Vitamin and mineral deficiencies are so prevalent, I want to do a few pages on the most frequent ones:

- *Vitamin B 12: This little supplement is really important, and does not stay in the body for a long time, it is water soluble, so you will not overdose. It does best if it is digested through the tissue in the mouth and throat, it is helped by having a lot of good bacteria in your digestive system. There is a book that everyone should read: Could it be the B12, it gives you so much information about how dangerous it is, if you do not have enough B12 in your body. One of the most dangerous things Is what it does to your brain, if you are deficient in B12 you can develop dementia, anemia, weakness, tiredness, rapid heart rate and rapid breathing pale skin, sore tongue, bruising, and disrupted bowel junction, constipation or diarrhea. If you are deficient for a long period you may develop symptoms of mental diseases. I believe that the medical world is not knowledgeable about how serious the problem becomes. Vegans and vegetarians are at risk because no B 12 in vegetables and they must supplement always. If your lab tests comes back low you must request further testing, "The Shilling Test".*

- *Vitamin C: A great many diseases can be "cured" with the use of this vitamin and if you take too much you will naturally discard it in your urine and it is a water soluble supplement. Sometimes massive doses of vitamin C is required by your body and since It is not very expensive everyone can take it. You may want to read some of Dr. Andrew Saul's books.. Iv vitamin C is given for many chronic diseases and especially in the treatment of cancer. To find our how much you need to take, take it until you start having diarrhea, you will then know the dosage you need to heal.*

- *B Complex group: If you have no energy, take a look at your intake of the B vitamins.   B complex contains Biotin, Riboflavin, Thiamine, Niacin, Pantothenic acid, Pyridoxine, Folic Acid and Cobolomine (B12)*

- *Vitamin D, not a vitamin but a hormone: There are many chronic diseases that many physicians believe are the result of not absorbing enough vitamin. I believe that part of this Is because we do not have enough cholesterol to absorb the sunshine that we do receive, which is not enough and when we are in the sun, we immediately shower it off our skin before we absorb it through our skin.*

- *Magnesium: I could speak for hours on our need for magnesium, it is the machine that runs most of the processes in our body, and is necessary for everything to work. Our food is deplete of magnesium because our soil is depleted so we must take it in a supplement and rub it on our bodies as an oil, cream or soaks.*

- *CoEnzyme Q 10:: Just a few years ago, research began to tell us how important this supplement is, until middle age or so, we make enough on our own, unless we are taking prescription drugs that deplete this cell energizer from our bodies. Because of the use of medication and our lifestyle, I believe that everyone over the age of 30 probably should take this supplement. It protects our cells and energizes every cell in our body.*

- *Potassium;:: such a great little need in our bodies: stimulates brain and nerve cells, stabilizes blood sugar, reduces muscle disorders, stabilizes blood pressure, regulates water balance, improves heart, bones and nerves, etc.*

There are others but these, in my opinion are the most prominent ones. Not only can you be deficient but you may lack the ability to absorb them, You must also concern yourself with the purity of the supplements you are purchasing.

Today I had a pedicure and haircut from a friend, a retired hairdresser and she continues to work doing pedicures for the elderly and disabled. After my pedicure my daughter took me for brunch, the waiter, an older man was really nice so I asked him about his job and he told me that he had not lived in town long and had been a farmer. I gave him a book of mine and ask him about what his ideal job was and I gave him my phone number so we could discuss his life's dreams at a later date. The brunch was sweet potato latke and I enjoyed it. I have such curiosity that I always am concerned that people are not happy in their job, I think that we should all be happy doing what we are doing.

New Chapter:

Since the health food store, where I had my classes and met clients closed this week, I had to find another spot to lead my classes. Yesterday I started teaching from a classroom in The First Christian Church in Rogers, Arkansas. The classroom is the best classroom I have had and I am hoping that attendance will increase so that I can keep teaching.   Since the store was closing, I spent lots of money on supplements for everyone but at a 70% discount, I did not spend too much, just had to think about who needed what.

Last weekend I signed up for the ACIM, Dr. Lee Cowden, conference, livestreaming on my computer. I missed some of the sessions and some that I really wanted, I missed because, my internet went down for some reason. I took notes but they are really hard to decipher because I was trying to write so many notes. A few of the speakers were not familiar to me so I had to do a bit of research. I am looking forward to a time and place to share all these great things that I am learning.

Dr. Calvin Bey informed me about the anti-aging machine, Bemer healing modality so I must "taste" that modality soon. I am also interested in Dr. Norm Shealy's new modality using crystals and scaler energy. Hearing Dr. Norm Shealy caused me to go back and relearn his acupuncture rings healing modality.

I had an invitation to check out a healthy lunch spot called: The Snack Lab, it was really a good place and had such things as bone broth, kefirs, etc. While ordering my lunch I met a lady who had a couple of businesses and learned some things from her. We also met the vendor/provider of the Kombucha, so learned from him and of course we had a long conversation with the owners of The Snack Lab, both the husband and wife. I love learning about local businesses especially if they are serving a niche and are creative.

Because today is Thanksgiving, I am imagining many households where there are one or two people who try to ruin everyone's day by being purest; "I don't eat sugar, I can't eat gluten", etc. etc. Please do not do this, find what you feel comfortable eating and don't speak! Unless you have a critical illness, your body can tolerate a bit of gluten, sugar, animal fat, or whatever, if you can't, make an excuse to stay home and go after the meal has been consumed. These problems are one reason I get upset with most vegans, they are so "pure" and self centered, they cannot let someone else enjoy themselves….just saying. Some people love their sensitivities so are not willing to work with people who can remove them: Ask and Receive, NAET, etc. You have to be willing to work with these modalities for healing.

What a week, Sunday, friends, left town and I got 2 large black lab dogs for the week, Gomer and Shadow come often so they have fun, Monday I had class with poor attendance then my daughter brought me a little chihuahua, his dad was homeless so the shelter took the dog. We got permission to take the dog until his dad found a place, a very frightened little dog who spent most of his time in my lap. Wednesday evening the dad got a bus ticket to go to relatives in California so the little boy went with him. Just as he left, 3 more large dogs came for the holiday and my little bity house is overfull. No space even to walk through the house but lots of love, dog kisses (saliva), and play. My own dogs and cats adjust but my little chihuahua, Heidi does not appreciate those big dogs getting my attention. This is my life, one of my daughters will take a bit of time from her jobs today and bring me, Thanksgiving dinner, probably a Pizza, since my whole family is having to work on the holiday. I have 3 dogs in my chair but am managing to write out some life planning plans for a few people and do some learning via my laptop. And audible is very valuable for learning when every animal wants a bit of attention.

Some of my favorite things:

- ➢ *Moringa:*
- ➢ *Black seed oil:*
- ➢ *Diatomaceous Earth:*
- ➢ *Goat milk Kefir:*
- ➢ *Noni Juice:*
- ➢ *Magnesium (Epson Salts):*
- ➢ *Coconut Oil:*
- ➢ *Eggs:*
- ➢ *Earthing:*
- ➢ *Cordyceps:*
- ➢ *Ashwanganda, Rhodiola, turmeric, Astragalus, Ginseng, Oil of oregano, olive leaf extract, Neem, dandelion, etc.*
- ➢ *Pets:*
- ➢ *Essential oils:*
- ➢ *Bone broth:*
- ➢ *Infrared, low level laser, PEMF,*
- ➢ *Castor Oil packs:*
- ➢ *Exercise, especially rebounding:*
- ➢ *Infared biomat*

A short life story

I must pause and relate something very personal, I have been told several times this year; I would love to live your life, I wish I had your life. Many people see the lives of others better than theirs and see the other people's lives without the problems. To tell you the truth, most people could not live my life, yet they see it as a perfect life.

I was living an average busy family life, I worked, my husband worked and all 4 children were doing well in school, then the bottom began to fall out, my husband lost his eyesight and we found that he had a brain tumor and after living with blindness for a year, he died. How could I pay for school for 4 children, help them live happy lives. Roy was 52 years old and I was 46. I felt alone and very sad, I knew that I must provide more income because my husband's teacher retirement paid out little more than his medical bills. When he became ill, I was administrator of a healthcare facility, it was a 24/7 job so I had to change, became a corporate nurse, a 40 hour week job. When he died I needed more income so added other jobs   As a perfect mom I needed to be a part of all the debate tournaments, musical recitals, etc. If you have been a young widow you know that all your social life changes because you have been friends with couples, you are no longer a couple so that changes also.

Just as I was becoming adjusted to being a single parent, I got a call at work that, my house was burning, it was one of those 3 story Victorian old homes full of "stuff" none of the stuff was important to anyone but me. I had a little house in another town so had some place I could live but it was not paid for so would be making monthly payments and my husband had not updated the insurance on our old home that burned so I needed to be making money, 2 children in college one in high school and one in junior high. We were given a dog to replace the dog that had died in the fire, what a gift, a puppy, we did not need. It was a little border collie puppy, the kids named him Oreo, he was black on each end white in the middle. Oreo was my emotional support for the next few years.

To make a long story shorter, I have struggled and worked for many years, I quit the medical nursing when I could no longer tolerate it and kept working so many jobs and learning everything I could about natural healing. I now live on social security less than $900 a month, live in a house that I do not have money to repair so have no working; garbage disposal, no working oven, no working dishwasher, no central heat and air, and I rescue animals; a dozen dogs, a couple of cats, a couple of elderly pigmy goats and a 36-year-old horse. As a child, I would be angry with all the adults in my world, I would remark, "when I grow up I am going to fill my house and yard with animals and completely avoid people". I have reached that goal. I can really mark that off my 'bucket list'.

My passion is helping people and pets, learning everything I can to help others. I have enough diplomas and certificates to paper the walls of this small house but I never feel that I have enough knowledge and I certainly will never learn how to make and keep money. I enjoy people and pets, therefore, I am happy every day, even though I struggle every day just to pay bills and keep myself well. Most 83 year old people live a different life and this is not the life I planned, I just had to take so many detours as I was trying to reach goals. But the only goals I needed were to be happy and well.

Now all those people who have money and nice homes, do they really want my life?

I believe that most often we think that there are "greener pastures on the other side". I have so much compassion for the homeless because, one lost check and I could be in their shoes. I am so grateful that since 1982, I have been able to keep my family and I from being homeless, given my children educational opportunities and helped many people.

I usually figure out a way to do the things on my bucket list, I have planned and produced a couple of Holistic Wellness Conferences, in the area. Great speakers and networking was great. The events did not make money but they were on my "bucket list".

Life Happenings

My husband and I met when both had very good professional careers, he was teacher and coach and I was an RN. When I became pregnant with our son we decided that we did not want *to raise a family in a city so looked at the map of the united states and found the area we wanted to raise our family and spent the spring break in the area applying for jobs with the school systems, we knew that I could work anywhere, in the field of nursing, I had made a high score on my boards so could go anywhere, start a job and get temporary license to work at any job in the field of nursing. He got job offers then we researched the school systems and small towns to find which job he would accept. That was not easy because the internet had not been born so no mrs. Google. We chose the town and we moved, using his teacher retirement from the state to use as a down payment on a little house. We lived in that small town, until his death and the house fire. A wonderful life for raising a family and becoming a part of the community. Because he was a teacher and athletic coach and I was a nurse, everyone knew us and our family, all 5000 people. We were also home of foreign students, on most of the boards for non profits and all 4 children had many opportunities for learning because we were less than an hour away from 4 colleges, etc. We went to the state legislature to promote the projects we believed in and made our voices heard.*

When I became homeless and responsible for the life and education of 4 children, I was feeling very defeated but I am a very stubborn lady and just kept moving one foot in front of the other, Even grabbing all the scholarships we could and me working 2 and 3 jobs, I have really never caught up financially. My children did grow up to be really nice people and I have kept myself very healthy, we have kept hitting speed bumps in life so never achieved any comfort, with money. I only use cash and a debit card so do not ever have debt, but struggle every month to have any of my social security check left at the end of the month.

I do realize that if I charged for my work, I could do better but, there are so many needs, I must say that all the workshops, seminars, etc. in managing finances and learning to charge for services, I have so many completion certificates, I could wall paper a wall. I am a "well educated" human because every job I have, I just have to be the best so I learn everything I can about what ever I am doing. As a Mary Kay beauty consultant, I never missed a learning opportunity, as a corporate nurse, I had to learn all about worker compensation and insurance, when I was a Pampered chef, I won every trip so I could take my children on vacations, I had friends who had a chain of restaurants so learned every job in the business, friends owned hotels, I learned the business so well that when they went on trips, I could stay in the hotel and oversee the business, working with the vo-tech education system and teaching the unemployed how to build a resume and get a job, was very interesting.

I loved selling Real Estate, I really enjoyed producing events and would still be doing that if a partner had not run it into bankrupt, Home nursing and dog sitting were easy to add to any job, as a nurse: nursing manager, administrator, teaching, etc. As an administrator of health care facilities, I became certified in dietary, physical therapy, activities director, social services assistant, occupational therapy and of course, the interaction with employees and patient's families was the largest learning curve. I had learned a lot of that because when my children were young I supervised day care and preschool programs. Earlier in my life I had also had all the Dale Carnegie classes and had made many speeches at the local clubs and at the colleges. I made the rounds to all the organizations when I had foreign students living with my family and when my husband and I were working trying to get day cares, foster homes etc. regulated in the state of Missouri. Everything I have done, in my opinion has been a great learning experience. I think I probably was the first person to listen to all the Tony Robbins tapes.

Several years ago, I spent a summer managing a horse ranch in Arizona, because my son needed me, I considered it a sabbatical. I also enjoyed working in retail customer service because I could be with people, I always either started an employee cookbook or a newsletter in the store. I had the opportunity to help open a Build A Bear store, A Kohl's and a Belk store, I have also opened 2 new Nursing homes.

I am so grateful that I have the opportunity to live in the computer age, it makes life so much more interesting.

More Learning:

Just listened to a webinar about the terrible things that happen when we have dental work and am reminded that I need to learn more so back to www.amazon.com for some Kindle books and an audible. As you probably know by now, I will not agree with everything I hear, I will do more research.

Every time I find a Kindle book that I am interested in reading, I start with the free sample and look at the table of contents. I will then have an idea of what is in the book and and will know if it will benefit my education. The theory that we are all alike and have the same needs is one of the worst belief systems promoted. I think that everyone has a unique body, mind and soul and we all have different needs, I never want anyone to be told what their body needs, we need to learn how to ask our bodies and how to treat the different needs. Most of us have very flexible bodies and we can tolerate a bit of sugar, dairy, gluten, etc. I know that my own body is very forgiving and when I do something foolish, it will take care of my problem without side effects. We are not made with cookie cutters and I am glad that I am unique. I really do not want to be like you!

New tips every day of what is out there to learn, just had a call about someone who healed his prostate cancer with cannabis. Saw another film on Theda energy healing, watched a seminar on stress management and I just downloaded the audible on "The obesity code" so much to learn and so little time.

Each time that I think I will close the book and publish, I start learning more and want to share. Last week was learning about the dangers of being an open mouth breather and the egoscue exercise program that shows how simple exercises can heal "sick" joints, then really got into the research on the Restore4life *product and am ordering more on Amazon. A couple of things that I need to do more study: essential oils, herbs, stem cells and cannabis.*

Today it is raining, I am sleepy and I don't really want to do anything that I need to do but must press on. I have been trying to switch my animals to a mostly homemade nutrition program, yesterday almost the whole day was consumed with; shopping, cutting meat, blending fruit and veggies and putting portions in the freezer. Not easy trying to do the right thing. I refuse to learn about a raw natural diet for my horse and goats. I have ordered a better daily supplement for the dogs and ordered a new supply of Willards Water for all the animals. I feel very good about the fact that it has been many years since I took any of my animals to the vet, never give them the worm or flea protection, no vaccines and they live long, happy lives. Supplements and diatomaceous earth are important for my animals, raw bones for my dogs and I sometimes give them bone broth and goat milk kefir. I also give my animals lots of love and freedom to be themselves, they also have access to outdoors in a large fenced yard at all times, 2 doggie doors and a cat door.

I love my electronics but sometimes I wish that I was better trained, I was trying to cut and paste and I lost a few pages that I wrote, I will probably find them when I am writing something else next month or next year. Monday for class I am preparing a group of 9 balloons and will write on the botom of each balloon a problem that is keeping us down and as we cut off the problem, our lives soar.

- *Procrastination and negative attitude: This is probably the number one thing that keeps us from reaching goals and living the ideal life, I just listened to an audible book "The 5 Second Rule", think of what you need to do and count down 5,4,3,2,1 and start. In another life I taught people the DIN. DIN method, do it now, do it now.*
- *Self centeredness: the people in this age seems to be getting more and more self centered, think of what you life is doing for others and adopt the "pay it forward" attitude.*
- *Judgmental: my oh my who appointed you the "holy judge" of others. I don't care what your beliefs are or what color you are, I accept you and your life without any question.*
- *Anger and Resentment: Some people spend their life being angry or should I say, they waste their lives. Release all anger swiftly and do not let resentment ruin your life.*
- *Lack of Wisdom: In the dictionary knowledge comes before success, it is so easy now to learn anything you need to learn and keep they brain of yours happy, so many opportunities for learning anything you want to learn.*
- *Unwillingness to change: Don't become stuck in your way and not open to changing. Be open to new ideas and if they benefit you, use them with delight, if not just let them pass or save for later use.*

- *Self worth: don't be afraid to be yourself, you are so unique. Just like a snow flake, you have a mission and ou are important for achieving that mission, only you are responsible for making yourself your very best self.*

Number 9 is reserved for the thoughts of the people in the class, each will write a problem that they want to be rid of and we attach to the balloon and let it go….let it go…let it go!

As I get ready to publish this book, it is difficult to wrap up. In the past few weeks, I have taken so many classes, seminars and webinars that gets me so excited about learning new things and have the ability to help so many more people. I have learned more about: metabolic syndrome (adult onset diabetes), healing cancer, preventing and healing dementias, using stemcell therapy, tapping to heal emotional problems, Ask and Receive treating, Essential oils benefits and healing disease, and many more. I learn something new every day and am fortunate that I have opportunities to learn. In my next booklet, I will have more and more to write about.

My Experts:

I have to share a list of the experts that I depend upon every day, for my extended learning, this is a partial list because there is not space for all my experts and you will want to add the experts along with contact information.

- ➢ *Dr. Josh Axe and Dr. Jordan Rubin*

- *.drlabrie@cox.net, Dr. LaBrie is a chiropractor that has added may healing modalities to her practice, including acupuncture, yoga, qigong*
- *Dr. Tom Cowan and Dr. Cowan's Garden*
- *Dr. Lee Cowden and ACIMconnect*
- *Dr. Stephen Sinatra*
- *Dr. Garry Gordon*
- *Dr. Joe Mercola: his interviews with experts on www.youtube.com*
- *Dr. Joan Vernikos: "Sitting Kills, Moving Heals"*
- *Dr. Andrew Saul*
- *Stephanie Seneff*
- *Dr. David Perlmutter*
- *Dr. Norm Shealy*
- *Dr. Ed Kondrot*
- *Bulletproof radio Dave Asprey @ Bulletproof com*
- *Dr. Carolyn Dean*
- *Dr. Kelly Brogan*
- *www.qigong.com*
- *Dr. Calvin Bey: Organic Gardening and Earth Energy*
- *Dr. David Tharp: Naturopath*
- *Robert Taylor: Tranquility Full Spectrum Health*
- *Teresa Jacobs- energy healing*
- *Biofeedback with Audrey Jared*
- *And many, many more. I can be contacted and I will connect you to some one who can help you.*

Blog: www.freddiemema.blogspot.com

e-mail: *freddiemema@hotmail.com*

Phone 479-366-4306

Questions?

Here are some questions to ask yourself, often:

Am I drinking pure water and staying hydrated?

Am I breathing pure, clean air and breathing deeply?

Have I developed an exercise program that I enjoy?

Am I practicing meditation?

Have I found the healers that are beneficial for my wellness and am I using them?

Do I learn new things every day?

Have I found a program to detoxify my body?

Have I replaced all prescription drugs with natural supplements or food?

Do I touch the earth daily?

Do I do something good for someone else every day?

Do I spend time laughing and playing every day?

Do I spend time socializing and meeting new people?

Have I deleted all the toxic hair products and cosmetics from my life?

Am I living a life of gratitude and forgiveness?

What am I doing every day that is bringing my life closer to that dream life?

Do I take responsibility for my problems or am I blaming someone or something for the problems, Do I take my power and use it?

I am certain that I am missing some questions and you are welcome to write all over this little book. There are other ideas in my other books and I would encourage you to read them.

More Life Coaching:

Take some time and write out your dreams and mission. You may want to make a dream poster, write a statement in your journal, 5,4,3,2,1, din, din. Start now making your life that dream life: body, mind and spirit.

- *Suggested wording to start your statement:*
- *I am living in ______working in ______and having so much joy and fun in my life----*
- *My financial success makes it possible for me to --------*
- *I have achieved wellness and no longer take drugs----*

Spend time working on positive statements to use in your statement of your dreams. These statements should be repeated often and celebrated when they are achieved.

I would suggest that you, de-clutter your home, your car, your calendar and your life. Only necessary appointments on your calendar, allowing time to do good deeds, laugh and play.

Make a bucket list, a list of things that you really want to do , and start marking things off as you do them. Do you want to travel, play or sing music, learn a language, meet someone, learn a new skill, etc. figure out how to do them at no cost, barter services or save money to accomplish your bucket list.

Do you want a better job, if you do, find out what you need to do to get that job; go back to school, learn another skill or write out why you can do the job and discuss it with your superior.

Look at a map and figure out where you want to live and start making plans to move, do your research and start writing out steps toward the move.

Make a list of things you enjoy doing then find out how you can use your spare time to volunteer your time to that organization.

One of the most important thing is to take time to plan and enjoy that phase of achieving your wants and needs. Sometime the journey is the most enjoyable part of the process.

If you are spending your time doing things you do not enjoy, (housekeeping, yard work, etc.) let someone else do it, if you have funds, you can hire someone and if you do not have the funds, barter the services.

Nothing can be accomplished if you don't put feet to your dreams. In other words, you must write out what you want and then steps to achieving those dreams. You may run into lots of detours or speed bumps but just keep making new paths and accomplish your dreams.

I find it easier if I use small notebooks for each thing I am working on such as, Plans for changing location: research where I want to live, how much would it cost to live there, cost of moving, if job is not portable research possibilities for employment, monthly income needed above present salary, date I want to move, purchase property or rent, etc.

Fail to Plan and You Plan to Fail!!

If you need help, enlist the assistance of friend or mentor or you may want a Life coach that you enjoy and barter the fees.

Let me remind you that there are mentors everywhere, find someone doing what you want to do and check to see if they might mentor you, if they turn you down, nothing lost, if they say yes, you gain a lot. A lot of retired people are just waiting to be ask to help you learn what they have already learned. In some cities there are retired organizations that want to help the younger generator learn. Your chamber of commerce has a list of volunteer organizations and also make friends with someone at the chamber because they can be a great asset for you. There was a time in my life when I was a member of 3 different chambers of commerce and found all very helpful. If you want to meet a lot of the business leaders of your community, purchase a ticket to their awards dinner, I would also recommend that you join your local chamber, if it is not too expensive.

Many, many years ago, I moved to a new city and my daughter went online finding the new businesses coming to town and I was fortunate to get in on the ground floor, helped set up the new business and was employed there until I moved again. At that time the internet was not as good as it is now, but we made good use of it.

Networking, networking, the most important thing to do, whether you want to change your job, change you living situation or just meet interesting people. If you want something, don't keep it a secret, tell everyone and you will make the connections you need. Several years ago, I went to a spring garden show at the gardens of my organic gardening teacher on May 2nd and it snowed, no one else came excepting one lady and as we were discussing the garden, we found that none of us really knew each other but we had such connections and her husband has been the healer that I refer most of my clients for Bowenwork.

Today I met a couple who was wanting to learn about wellness and it was an accidental connection. You never know who will bring you a connection to a need that you have or a need that an acquaintance may have. I will admit that I am a very curious person and ask questions of everyone because I want to know about them and their wants and needs. Talking and listening are very important.

Every few months we need to reevaluate our life plan and tweak it so that it fits our needs. As you meet new people and learn new things we should change many of those wants and needs again this is where you need a life coach or a mentor. The reevaluation is a great fun and learning experience and we need to make it fun, keeping your journal up to date will assist you in making the correct tweaks to your life program.

To be continued……..

If you need assistance e-mail or text me: 479-366-4306 freddiemema@hotmail.com

www.ingramcontent.com/pod-product-compliance
Lightning Source LLC
Chambersburg PA
CBHW081853250726
48659CB00008B/2723